Made in the USA
Monee, IL
08 May 2022

96100132R00057